MW01298010

C-BAT
for
Parents
of
ADHD Children

Cognitive-Behavior Attention Training for Use by Parents of Attention Deficit and Attention Deficit Hyperactive Children

DR. JOHN N. MARR

ISBN: 1500751146
ISBN 13: 9781500751142
Library of Congress Control Number: 2014914264
CreateSpace Independent Publishing Platform,
North Charleston, South Carolina 29414

TABLE OF CONTENTS

CHAPTER 1

Introduction

This manual presents a special program to help parents with their children who have attention problems. The program introduced in this book has been proven to improve attention at home and at school.

These parents of the ADHD child are burdened with extra work and need help. The demands of an ADHD child can be physically exhausting and psychologically exhausting because of the need to monitor the child's activities and actions. And these behaviors and the parent's knowledge of the consequences of those behaviors make the parent anxious and stressed. The child's inability to "listen" is frustrating. The frustration often leads to anger and that anger often makes the parent feel guilty.

Lets first take a closer look at the characteristics of these children. If your child has been diagnosed as having Attention Deficit Disorder (ADD) or Attention Deficit Hyperactivity Disorder (ADHD), it is because he or she met the criteria of the American Psychiatric Association. These criteria are listed in the diagnostic manual of the American Psychiatric Association (1994). Those children and adolescents have at least six of the following symptoms,

1) often fails to give close attention to details or makes careless mistakes in schoolwork or other activities.

2) often has difficult sustaining attention in tasks or play activities.

3) often does not seem to listen when spoken to directly.

4) often does not follow through on instructions and fails to finish schoolwork, chores, or duties (not due to being oppositional or failure to understand).

5) often has difficulty organizing tasks and activities.

6) often avoids, dislikes or is reluctant to engage in tasks that require sustained mental effort (such as schoolwork or homework).

7) often loses things necessary for tasks or activities (toys, school assignments, pencils, books, or tools).

8) is often easily distracted by extraneous stimuli.

9) is often forgetful in daily activities.

Although those are defining symptoms, the diagnosis is confirmed by the intensity, persistence, and clustering of these symptoms rather than their presence or absence (Ross & Ross, 1982). The children and adolescents who demonstrate these clusters of symptoms experience serious problems in school and as many as half of them also show the characteristic defiant behaviors of oppositional disorder at home. However, children who only meet some of the symptoms also have serious attention problems at school and at home. In our experience these children want help.

Treatments

Medication is the most common treatment of ADHD. Medicines for treatment of ADHD are categorized into stimulants and non stimulants. Common stimulant medications are Adderall, Concerta, Vivanse, and Focalin. These medication help the child focus his thoughts and ignore distractions. They are effective in 70 to 80% of cases. They bring about a fast change in the childrens

behavior. Side effects are uncommon and when they occur, they usually last for just a few days. The most common side effects are loss of appetite, sleep problems, and headaches, The side effects can be eliminated by adjusting the dosage, changing the schedule of medication, or taking a different medication. Among the non stimulant medications are Intuniv and Straterra. Those medicines can help with impulse control and concentration.

It is important to know that medication will bring about the fastest change of any types of treatments but that the medication brings about no permanent change. If the child is taken off the medication, he will revert back to the previous state of problems in attention and concentration.

The new treatment for ADHD is a psycho-social approach that has been developed across the last 20 years. It is called Cognitive-Behavioral Attention Training (C-BAT). In the rest of this manual we introduce you to this training which you can began to use immediately. By the way, C-BAT can be used with or without medication.

Every procedure in C-BAT is directed at making the child use the executive function of his brain which is what these children fail to do. It characterizes them; they don't use the executive function of their brains. It is this function which is located in the frontal lobe of the brain and which children, adolescents, and adults with attention deficit disorder don't use. The executive function includes the management of time and attention, allows one to switch focus, plan and organize, remember details, curb inappropriate speech or behavior, and allows one to integrate past experience with present action. Chapters 2 through 9 tells you, the parent, how to use procedures that train the child to use his or her executive function.

Some of the types of problems reported by parents of ADHD children are shown in Table 1. This checklist will allow you to compare his behaviors now with what he is like after you have used the procedures described in this book.

3

Table 1
Check off those that characterize your child or adolescent

1._____ does not have the necessary materials even when told of the need ahead of time.

2.__✓__ says she has lost the materials and doesn't know where they are.

3._____ can't find completed assignments.

4.__✓__ can't find personal possessions.

5.__✓__ does not follow the required steps of the assignment, seems to have skipped or not noticed some steps.

6.__✓__ watches others instead of his work.

7._____ in school does not complete the assignment during class time.

8._____ sits and does nothing.

9.__✓__ in school has to be placed at front of room because of distractions.

10.__✓__ says he didn't understand the assignment.

11.__✓__ gets out of seat a lot at home or school.

12.__✓__ acts silly or makes funny noises to get attention at home or school.

13.__✓__ doesn't listen to directions.

14.__✓__ doesn't follow directions

15.__✓__ makes careless mistakes.

16._____ fails to complete homework.

17._____ completes homework but doesn't turn it in.

18.__✓__ seems to have difficulty in organizing self to get started on task.

19.__✓__ avoids or dislikes activities that require sustained work or attention.

20.__✓__ fiddles with material in desk, pocket, or purse when the teacher is talking or when he is supposed to be working.

CHAPTER 2

Self Control

As was said in the last chapter many of the ADHD children have been raised in home environments where there were no consequences for not paying attention. To put it another way, if you never have been without food, you don't worry about having food. If you have never fallen down, you don't have to watch where you walk, run, or climb. If you have never been cold, you don't have to remember to wear a coat or remember where you put it. Many of these children who have attention problems were raised by great care-giving parents. And to compound the problem of the parents who are always doing things for their children, or picking up after them, the parents do not have a lot of time or patience. Today in our society there are millions of homes where we have two very busy adults who have time consuming and important jobs and where the parents have learned that it is easier to do things for the child than to teach the child to do it himself.

"Johnny, put on your shoes." Later, "Did you put on your shoes?" No answer. Parent goes and looks. "Hurry up or we're going to be late. Oh, come here, I'll put them on for you."

Did Johnny have to pay attention? No. What the parents say in these circumstances is just noise to the child because there are no consequences for listening or not listening, for doing or not doing. Correcting the problem can become even more difficult if the child finds that consequences are provided some of the time and not delivered at other times. Furthermore, there is no way for

5

the child to predict when there will be consequences for not paying attention or for doing what one was told to do.

A Need for Self Control

Regardless of how he got that way, we do know that the student doesn't pay attention as demonstrated by those 20 behaviors listed in the check list in the first chapter. Children who have attention problems are sometimes said to lack a sense of responsibility or lack self-control. The characteristic choices made by those who lack self control are shown in Table 2.

Table 2
The Person who Lacks Self Control

1. Chooses behaviors that have immediate small reinforcers even thought this will result in later big punishers.

2. Chooses behaviors that have immediate small rewards rather than behaviors that have delayed big rewards.

3. Chooses behaviors that avoid immediate small unpleasantness even though there will be delayed rewards if they don't avoid the temporary unpleasantness..

4. Chooses to avoid small unpleasantness that is immediate even though this will result in delayed strong punishers or much unpleasantness later.

If we examine the behaviors of students who have problems with attention, we find that every one of the behavioral problems associated with a lack of attention and shown in Table 1 can be analyzed in terms of the self-control characteristics.

Among the signs of attention difficulties is Number 6 in Table 1, **the student who watches other students instead of the teacher, board, or book.** This behavior is an example of the first

characteristic of individuals lacking in self-control, choosing small immediate reinforcement despite the fact that it results in a delayed strong punisher. It is fun to watch the other kids right now. The consequence for not watching the teacher is delayed. He does not get the poor grade until much later. Similarly Number 20 in Table 1, **fiddles with material in desk, pocket, or purse when the teacher is talking or when he is supposed to be working,** is another example of the first characteristic of individuals lackin g in self-control. It is more fun to fiddle with materials in one's pockets than to listen to the teacher or read the book. The consequence doesn't come until much later.

Another type of failure of self-control is the second characteristic of choosing immediate small reinforcement over delayed larger reinforcers as illustrated in this example, **does not complete the assignment during class time.** He doesn't complete his classwork because he is **fiddling with material in desk, pocket, or purse when the teacher is talking or when he is supposed to be working,** or because of **finding excuses to leave her work, seat, or the room.** As a result she misses the play time during recess because she must finish her classwork.

One activity that fits the third characteristic of those who lack self-control is the habit of avoiding immediate punishers even though they are small with the result the student will not receive delayed reinforcers. Thus he is seen **getting out of his seat a lot at home and at school.** For him sitting there is punishment even though it is not that bad. As a result of his not staying in his seat, he doesn't get to do something later that is fun such as watching TV.

And examples that fit the criteria of the fourth characteristic of students who lack self-control, avoiding immediate small unpleasantness even though it results in delayed larger unpleasantness, is Number 16 in Table 1, his **failure to complete homework,** and Number 19, **avoiding or disliking activities that required sustained work or attention.** Because he is avoiding the homework

or activities that require work, he will get poor grades or even a tongue-lashing.

We need to teach these children self-control and to do this we need to use a variety of techniques. But each is aimed at training the child to pay attention and use their executive functions of their brains. Let's start with some new ways to use positives.

CHAPTER 3

How to Do It with Positive Reinforcement

The most powerful method of changing children's behaviors or creating those behaviors that are important in everyday life at home or at school is through the use of positive reinforcement. It can be used to produce new behavior, to increase behaviors that the child does occasionally, and to replace inappropriate behaviors with more desirable behaviors.

Just about everybody believes they know what positive reinforcement is and how to use it but most of the time they have some misunderstanding. Positive reinforcement is not the same as a reward. Positive reinforcement is actually anything that follows a behavior and increases the probability of that behavior occurring in the future. Certainly a candy or even a soda pop can be given as reinforcement but other examples include the sound of music, a touch, seeing a picture, a smile. Sometimes even a sound, a sight, or even an action that is unexpected, all will act as reinforcement. The test of its reinforceability is whether the behavior it is meant to reinforce increases in frequency. If "please" by the child is followed by something the child wants, "please" increases in frequency in the future when the child wants something.

Even behavior can be used to reinforce other behavior. "If you pick up your toys, you can go outside and play." The rule is that any behavior that is higher in probability can be used to reinforce a behavior that is lower in probability. Children would rather watch

TV than feed and water the dog. Watching TV is a high probability behavior and feeding the dog is a low probability. So watching TV should be allowed only after the dog is watered and fed. How often do we hear children and adolescents say I'll do it as soon as this program is over? We know that after that program is over they will find some other program to watch or something else to do other than feeding the dog. The rule for the parent has to be to tell them to feed the dog and then they can watch TV.

In one classroom, a teenage girl didn't want to do anything that the others wanted to do. She wasn't interested in visiting with girlfriends, reading the teen magazines, going to the library or even going outside during recess. All she wanted to do was sit in her chair in the classroom. Since sitting in the chair was a high probability behavior for her, it could be used to reinforce any of the other behaviors or even doing homework. She was informed that for every 15 minutes of reading a book in the library, looking at a magazine, or talking and listening to other students, she could sit in the chair in the room for 15 minutes. This requirement soon began to cause her to interact with others. She learned that interacting with others was more fun than just sitting in the classroom chair doing nothing.

One phrase that should not be used to reinforce is "Thank you" because thank you means that the child has done something for us. It should not be used when the child is doing something that he or she is supposed to do such as sitting in their seats quietly or putting their books away when directed. Parents should not say "Thank you" when the child hangs up his coat when he comes in the house, puts away his toys, or picks up his dirty clothes and puts them in the basket or hamper.

Instead the parent or teacher can say "that's great", "good job", "You are playing well with your sister" "You put those toys away without me telling you", "right on", "excellent", "give me a high five", "atta girl", "tremendous", Even a wink or a smile can act as a reinforcement.

One of the ways I have helped parents learn the power of re-inforcement is through the use of **Differential Reinforcement of Other Behavior (DRO)** to decrease a problem behavior. The name sounds like something very complicated but it really is a simple technique for parents to follow. I ask the parents to watch for an occasion when they are talking in a room and the child comes into that room. The parents are asked to stop talking immediately and say to the child, "We are talking and you have not interrupted us once. That is great. Is there anything you need to say to us before we continue talking?" The child is likely to look quite surprised because he had not even noticed that they were talking. Similarly, when the parent answers the phone, they again should try DRO. "Hello. Hi, How are you. Could you hold on a moment?" Then the parent puts their hand over the phone and says to the child, "I'm on the phone and you have not interrupted me. That is great. Is there anything you need to say to me before I go back on the phone?" This is a much more successful way of teaching children not to interrupt than just telling them not to interrupt.

When you see that the child is inhibiting himself from inter-rupting, you can began to delay the reinforcement for not inter-rupting by waiting longer and longer to reinforce. But don't drop it entirely. At first you are reinforcing every time you are on the phone or when he enters a room where you are in a conversation with another. Then you can move to every second time and then back to every time, then every third time and then about every fourth time. Soon you don't have to reinforce that behavior at all. And we are teaching him self-control and to pay attention. You really don't have to count how often you reinforce but just remem-ber to thin out the reinforcement by giving it less frequently. We examine the use of partial reinforcement in a later chapter.

We are teaching them behavior – consequence, behavior- con-sequence, appropriate behavior – positive consequence. But when the behavior is inappropriate – negative consequence. Positive is

not enough. Discipline must also occur. Let's take a look at that in the next chapter.

CHAPTER 4

Discipline for Attention

We know that the child does not have to take responsibility for her behavior if there never or hardly ever are any consequences. We saw that in the Chapter on Self-Control. She can do what she wants and does not have to pay attention to what the consequences are for the behavior. We pay attention to our speed when we are driving our cars and the posted signs on the streets because there can be expensive consequences if we speed.

In addition to the problem of a lack of self control there are problems created by children who are oppositional. A large percentage of children who have ADHD have also been found to have the diagnosis of Oppositional Defiant Disorder. They refuse to do what they are told and in some cases openly defy their parents.

The discipline procedure that we recommend is Time Out (TO). But it is my type of Time Out. I have had parents tell me, "Oh, we have tried Time Out and it doesn't work", and I tell them that if they use Time Out the way I describe, it will work. When the child misbehaves, he is told exactly what it is that he did. "You were told not to throw the ball in the house but you continued doing it. You are now going to have a Time Out as a result. The child is directed to sit on a TO pillow within sight of the parents and out of sight of the television. A timer is started for 7 minutes. The timer is across the room from the child. If the child refuses to go into TO, he is sent to his room until he is ready to go into TO. If he refuses to go, the parent takes him by the arm and hurries him to his room and says "Stay there until you are ready to

go to TO. When he finally agrees The timer is started and if the child talks or calls the dog, the clock is restarted to 7. If again he talks, the clock is restarted and he is told this is his last chance. If he again talks, sings, or gets off the pillow, he is told that he is not ready for his TO and must go to his room for 15 minutes. When the timer rings at 15 minutes, he is asked if he is ready to go into Time Out. If he says, "No", the clock is set for another 15 minutes. If he comes out in two minutes and says he is now ready, the parent says, "No, you said you weren't ready so I have restarted the clock for another 15 minutes. When the clock rings again, I will again ask you if you are ready for TO. That extra 15 minutes seems like an eternity for children when they want outside their room. Never again will he say that he's not ready. So when he says he is ready, he is told to come out and go sit on the TO pillow. The timer is reset to seven minutes and when it rings, the parent is instructed to tell him again why he is in TO and that the next time he acts that way he will again have a TO.

Remember, we are trying to be consistent. We want him to pay attention to his own behavior. And not just when he is at home.

Once a child has been placed in time out for a specific behavior, i.e. hitting, he should not be given warnings in the future for that behavior. Parents too often say, "Remember what happened to you last week when you were hitting". After a while the child comes to depend upon the parent's warning to tell him when not to do something instead of learning to control his own behavior. We want him to pay attention to his own behavior.

It is helpful if the TO is recorded in a notebook. You can see how the Time Outs are occurring less often, what he is going into Time Outs for, and that you have to restart the clock less often. When recording, TO means he went into TO and you did not have to restart the clock. RTO means he refused to go into TO and you had to send him to his room until he was ready to go to the TO place. TO2 means you had to restart the clock once. TO3 means

you had to restart it two times. TO3RTO means you had to send him to his room and then he came out and did TO.

Applications of Time Out

At the Dinner Table. Children often have difficulty settling down to eat after being called from playing. They still want to play, tease, and have fun. This includes grabbing their brother's utensils or even food, throwing food, grabbing for dishes in order to be first, opening the mouth wide when it is filled with food to "gross out" their sister, and even bringing toys to the table. Parents have to have firm rules about behavior at the table or else dinner time becomes chaos. Some parents have just about given up having a family dinner and just let the kids come to the table or into the kitchen to get their food and take it back in front of the TV. If the children see that the parents mean it when they give a dinner table rule, they soon will began to settle down and follow the rules.

Table Time Out:

1. Tell the child what he did that was inappropriate. Be specific. "For grabbing the bread away from your brother". Tell the child to put his utensil down on the table, put his hands in his lap, be still, and take time out from the dinner for 30 seconds. At the end of the half minute, he can resume dinner.

2. Make it clear that if he can't be still for a half minute time out at the table, he will be sent to the regular Time Out place for a regular Time Out. At the end of the regular Time Out the child is allowed to come back to the table to resume his meal.

In a Restaurant. The same two step process is used as at the dinner table at home. **If the child misbehaves at the table, she is**

first given a chance to take her 30 seconds quietly at the table. If she continues to misbehave, she is escorted outside to the car and takes her regular Time Out there. Because being escorted out to the car is so embarrassing to them, children almost never will test this rule if they are told that is what will happen. Good behavior in the restaurant should be praised and, sometimes, rewarded.

In a Store or Mall. Children should be told **before** they enter the store or the mall that misbehavior will not be tolerated and that Time Out will be used if necessary. After being told and shortly after they enter the store, the parent should tell them that their behavior is appropriate and praise them. Frequent praise of staying close, not nagging for candy, toys, or clothes heads off a lot of misbehavior. Misbehavior is quickly dealt with. The young child is told to hold onto the cart or the parent's hand for 30 seconds because of the misbehavior. If he refuses or continues to misbehave, he is escorted out to the car and given a 3- 7 minute time out and told again what his misbehavior was. At the end of the time out period he is again told what he did that was wrong and that he will be given another time out if he misbehaves again.

Sometimes parents say that this type of discipline is too time consuming. My response is that they will save time in the future because the child will quickly learn that appropriate behavior is approved and sometimes rewarded but that misbehavior always has a Time Out consequence.

In the Car Misbehavior in the car is not unusual. Children have just got out of school and are excited about going home and having fun, or are on their way to school and don't want to go. They are more likely to misbehave when there are siblings in the car than when they are alone with the parent.

If the inappropriate behavior is for teasing, hitting, slapping, kicking, etc., the parent has a choice of having the child pay the time out by 1) delaying the trip home 2) demanding a time out in the car or 3) providing a time out when they get home.

1. Delaying as a Time Out. When children are in a hurry to get home, they don't want a delay of 5 minutes. The parent informs the children about the consequence for inappropriate behavior. If their fighting or arguing continues, the parent says, we will take a 5 minute time out and pulls the car over to the side of road (if it is safe to stop there) or into a parking lot and parks for five minutes. Tell the children that the time does not begin until they are quiet. It helps if the parent has something to do during that time such as reading a book or knitting, etc. At the end of the Time Out, the parent again tells them why the Time Out occurred and that another will occur if that inappropriate behavior occurs again.

2. Time Out in the Car This procedure demands that the child sit still and not talk for 5 to 7 minutes. It also requires that the parent monitor the child to see that he does sit still and not play during that time. If the parent can not do that and the child can not be trusted to sit still, then this type of Time Out should not be used.

During the national drive to solicit money to help in the restoration of the Statute of Liberty, they showed many television shots of the Statue from many angles during that summer. One mother told me that her 5 year old boy did something inappropriate in the car and so she told him he would have to take time out "Right Now". She added "Real Still. Just like a statue". A minute later she looked in the rear view mirror and saw him staring straight ahead, very still, and his arm in the air just like the statue of liberty.

3. Bridge When the parent doesn't have the time to pull the car over, he or she can use a Bridge. This is a card with the word "TIME OUT" printed in big black or red letters. It can be kept in the glove compartment or in a purse. When the behavior in the car is unacceptable, the parent informs the children to stop the behavior and if they do not stop, the parent pulls the card out and sets it on the dash board or on the seat and informs them that they have just earned a Time Out when they get home. The

card bridges the delay between the incident and the driving time to the home. The bridge works better than just telling the child that he will have to pay a Time Out. The card stays there when words are soon forgotten. Children soon learn that they better listen to the parent in the car or they are going to pay the price of disobedience.

In the Morning or When the Family is Leaving the House. Sometimes a parent will report that they don't have time to put the child in time out because they are in such a hurry to get somewhere that they will be late if they take the time to put the child in Time Out, especially when they are in a hurry to get the children to school and then to get to work on time. Putting the child in Time Out in the car usually will not be effective because he has to get in the car any way and probably doesn't want to go to school that day anyway. But using a bridge on a magnet on the refrigerator works very well. The card signifies that when the child gets back to the house, after school or whatever, and before he can watch television or go out to play, he will have to spend some time in Time Out.

During one visit I recommended this procedure to some parents when they had described how their very bright 4 year old knew that they had to hurry in the morning to get to work. They had reported that overall his disobedience and tantrums and refusals had decreased to near zero except on those mornings when he had to go to nursery school and they had to go to work. He then refused to turn off TV, get dressed, or come to the breakfast table. He called them names and said "I won't" or "I don't have to". We knew that he liked to go to nursery school, and I questioned them to make sure they were continuing to praise him when he did do the things they asked.

On their next visit two weeks later, he came marching into my office ahead of his parents and said, "Dr Marr, I'm mad at you." I said "Why are you mad at me?" With a very angry look on his face

he replied," Because you are the one who told them to start putting that Time Out Card up on our refrigerator." I said but that is
only to be used when you don't do what you're told" He replied, "I
don't care. They should have to think of these things themselves
and you shouldn't tell them." His parents told me that after the
first couple of times that they put that card up and on one morning put two cards up, the problem behaviors all but disappeared.
During the first week they had put it up and made him pay the
delayed Time Out on three mornings but this week they had only
had to put it up on one morning, today, which is one reason why
he was so mad. He was going to have to take a 4 minute Time Out
when he got home.

In most cases a delay in the time out can not be used until the
child is 5 years or older because the Bridge does not work as well
for the younger child.

At the Grandparent's or at a Friend's House. When the child
misbehaves at the grandparent's or at a friend's house, it is very
important that he discover that the rules remain the same. If the
parent does not use the same consequence, the child will quickly
learn that he can do as he wishes without consequences when he is
away from home. It is better to use an immediate consequence of
time out but, in some instances, immediate time out is not possible
and a delayed time out is then used.

It is important that the child be informed that Time Out will
be used. The place for Time Out should also be described and,
in some cases, parents do as I do in my office and ask the child
for ideas on where a good place for Time Out will be. Parents
are amazed how their children will help select a place for Time
Out. Of course, the grandparents or friends should also be fore-
warned and asked ahead of time if that is going to be a problem
for them. In all cases the children and grandparents and friends
should be reassured that you do not expect to have to use Time
Out. .

Time Out from Activities

When we remember that Time Out means the loss of opportunity to earn positive reinforcement, it is understandable that having to sit on a chair for a few minutes and do nothing and not be able to see anything of interest is the loss of reinforcement ---- the loss of the opportunity to do fun things.

In the adult world, time out includes jail time or house arrest. And juvenile delinquents are sometimes sentenced to some kind of "lock down". In prisons, convicts who misbehave are sometimes placed in solitary confinement where they can not go outside for exercise or use such privileges as the prison library, and they get time out from having visitors.

But another form of Time Out for children and adolescents is to remove the fun activities rather than send the child to a Time Out place. Examples are,

a. When brother and sister are fighting over the channel in stead of choosing to take turns, the TV is turned off for fifteen minutes or half an hour.

b. When the 4 year old throws sand, he must leave the sand box for 4 minutes, which to him seems like the rest of his life.

c. When the siblings continue to argue over a game, they have to stop playing it for a period of time. The period should be short, like 10 minutes, so they have an opportunity to practice the appropriate behavior by playing again.

d. The basketball coach makes the player, who swore, sit out of practice for 10 minutes.

e. The 7 year old must come in from playing outside because of misbehavior in the back yard or because he left the yard without permission.

Notice the time out periods are short. No basketball for 10 minutes, so that the player gets an opportunity to be back in the game and receive praise for the correct behavior. The players learn to practice good behavior in order to continue playing.

Grounding is another form of Time Out. To be grounded from TV, is the loss of opportunity to receive the pleasure of watching TV.

To be grounded from the use of the phone is the loss of opportunity to receive the pleasure of talking with one's friends.

Trouble Shooting Time Out

What do you do if he won't go to Time Out?

Answer: Send him to his room until he says he is ready to go into time out. Usually that is not long. But sometimes children who have been having their own way for a couple of years seem to want to show that they are boss and don't have to go. Some will even fall asleep. If he sleeps through the night, send him back to his room when he gets out of school the next day.

If his room is a place where he likes to go because of all the toys, tv, or computer there, then send him to a different room until he is ready to do a Time Out.

What do you do if he acts like he likes to be in Time Out?

Answer. Stay with the plan and continue the Time Out procedure. In a couple of days he will begin to act like he doesn't like it.

What do you do if he wants you to restart the clock, and will even get off the Time Out Pad to make you restart it?

Answer. Stay with the procedure and he will get tired of the clock and begin trying some other method of getting out of Time Out.

Remember, we are teaching the child to use his executive function to overcome attention problems. He does not have to pay attention to what he is doing if there are no consequences for his behavior. But when consequences are consistent he begins to

have to think about his behavior and the consequences. When he does that, he is beginning to use the executive function part of his brain.

CHAPTER 5

Self Talk

One of the major characteristics of children with attention deficit disorder is that they do not talk to themselves about what they are doing or about what they are supposed to do. They usually rely on their parents or teachers to remind them about what they should be doing, what they need to remember to do, or what is going to happen if they do forget.

Meichenbaum has referred to parents as Metacognitive Processing Prosthetic Devices. Metacognitions: thoughts about self and abilities. Metacognitive Processing: applying what one knows about ones self, i.e. what do I need to remember before I leave for school. Prosethetic Device: Like a crutch.

A mother who constantly reminds her child what he needs to do is acting as a Metacognitive Processing Prosthetic Device.

"Don't forget to hang up your wet towel." "Don't forget to bring your book home from school." "Don't forget to put your homework in your backpack." "Don't forget to take your glass into the kitchen."

If we can teach the child to talk to himself about what he needs to do and not do, what he must not forget, and when he should do things, he will be much better at remembering and doing those things he needs to complete.

Talking and Memory

Learning to verbalize about what we are doing takes effort. It is not easy to talk about what we are doing. But the effort we make is important to helping us to remember. Some people are in the

habit of walking around and talking to themselves. They report having whole conversations sometimes. Interesting enough we have found that those people are more intelligent.

We have three memory stages. The first is Sensory Memory which only lasts a few seconds. We see something and what we see is gone almost immediately unless we convert the sensory memory into something that is stored in Short Term Memory which is also called Working Memory. Once something is received in short term memory we can hold onto it by rehearsing it, or working on it. The more we work on the information that we received from sensory memory, the longer we can hold it in memory. We can began to store it in Long Term Memory by repeating it, by working on it, by rehearsing it, and even by writing it down.

If you write down what was said in the previous paragraph, you are working on the information. You will find that the effort of recording it on paper also caused it to begin to store it into long term memory.

Similarly, when we have the child talk about the math problems or mathematical symbols, we are teaching him how to store information about mathematics into long term memory. The more the child is made to work at verbalizing and relating the material to something that is already known, the more the material is being stored into long term memory where it can be retrieved later. "What does that addition (or multiplication) remind you of? How do you suppose addition helps people? How does it help in stores and in building something?"

Another major way we teach children to talk to themselves is through Self- Instructional Training. This procedure was first used by two psychologists,

Meichenbaum and Goodman (1971). Here it is.

1. An adult model performed a task while talking to himself out loud (cognitive modeling).

This would mean in our case that the parent talks to herself out loud about what she should do if she was the child.

2. The student performed the same task under the direction of the model's instructions (overt, external guidance). This means that we would have the child say the same things as the parent did with help from the parent.

3. The student performed the task while instructing himself aloud (overt self-guidance). This means we would have our child do the same thing while talking himself through it.

4. The student whispered the instructions to himself as he went through the task (faded, overt self guidance). Thus we have the child whisper to himself the same instructions as he does the task.

5. The student performed the task while guiding his performance via private speech (covert self-instruction). This time he does it again but doesn't make any sound.

Let's apply it to homework. Although we will look in depth at their doing their homework in a later chapter, the first thing we have to get them to do is to make sure they get the correct homework assignment. So if we apply self instructional training to homework, we would start out with the situation of imagining that he is sitting in the classroom and the Teacher is telling everybody to copy down the homework assignment. The parent says "What should you do? You should pull out your notebook and copy down the assignment the teacher makes. Is that a good thing to do? Yes because you will know what the assignment is when you get home. Then you can do the homework and turn it in. Who will be happy then? Your teacher, your parents and you." Notice that the parent asks all the questions and gives the answer to each.

Then as listed in the rules of Self Instruction, you start over but this time your child must answer the questions. If he can't answer, you give him the answer and start all over, "Pretend that the teacher is telling everybody to copy down the homework. What should you do?" The parent pauses and waits for the child to answer. If the child doesn't say "Pull out my notebook and copy down the assignment", the parent gives him the answer and has him say it. But since you had to give him the answer, you start all over. "Pretend that the teacher says, alright everybody copy down the homework assignment. What should you do?" When he says "Pull out my notebook and copy down the assignment", the parent says "Great. Is that a good thing to do?" and when the child says, "Yes", the parent says "Why is that a good thing to do?" and if the child doesn't answer, the parent gives him the answer and starts all over again.

When he can answer all the questions, then he must do it again, but this time he must ask and answer the questions. Thus, he must ask "What should I do?" And then answer that and ask the next question, "Is that a good thing to do?" "Yes, why is it a good thing to do?" After answering that question, we then have him do the whole thing in a whisper, and then again only moving his lips. Then finally saying it to himself. This type of exercise tells him that you will not let him escape doing the correct homework, and then turning it in. He is also learning to talk to himself.

Remember we are trying to get the children to use the executive part of their brains. They do this when they talk about what they are doing. They are also able to remember better when they talk to themselves about what they are doing. The more they tell you about what they are doing the more they are using the executive part of their brains.

We can use self- instructional training also to hang up clothes, to put her shoes away when she takes them off, and to set the table without being asked. Meanwhile we must be prepared to reinforce her successes.

CHAPTER 6

Over Correction Positive Practice

Positive Practice is a very useful procedure in training children to better pay attention. Typically they leave their dirty clothes laying on the floor when they take them off instead of putting them in the hamper as they have been taught. Similarly, they don't pay attention to where they took off their shoes in the house so that the next morning they are hunting all over to find the shoes so they can get ready for school. Or they leave their bikes laying on the front lawn where they can be stole rather than putting them in the car-port or garage when they are through riding them.

To teach them to pay attention to these acts when they occur we need to teach them that there is a consequence to their inattention. Positive practice means that the child will have to practice doing the right behavior whenever he does the wrong behavior. Over correction means that he will have to do it a number of times. Although longer and longer periods of Time Out do not have much effect on misbehavior, more and more positive practices have been found to be helpful in teaching a child the correct behavior. The first time he must practice 3 times, the next 4, the next 5, etc.

Example 1:

Johnny takes his clothes off in the bathroom before he takes his bath or shower and does not put them in the hamper before he leaves the bathroom.

Parent: "Johnny come back into the bathroom. You left your clothes on the floor instead of putting them in the

hamper. Pick them up and put them in the hamper." Johnny does it after complaining. Parent: "Good. But since you didn't do it in the first place, you need practice putting them in the hamper. Take them out of the hamper and put them back on the floor." Much complaining but he does it. Parent: "Now put them in the hamper"

When he does it, the parent says, "Good. Now you need to practice it one more time." When he does it, the parents says, "That's the way you should do it every time you take your dirty clothes off in here. The next time you leave them on the floor will mean that you need more practice."

Example 2

Mary takes her shoes off in the living room and leaves them there when she goes to her room at night. Parent: "Mary come back into the living room. You left your shoes here even though you have been told many time to take them to your room. You need practice. Take them to your room, put them down (or away) and then bring them back. Do that 3 times." After she has done it, "Good, the next time you leave them in the living room, I will again have you practice but since three times did not produce a change, we will practice four times."

Over-correction positive practice has been successful in treating many problem behaviors. In my clinical practice parents have reported that they have found it to be successful with the following,

Not making the bed before they leave for school. When this is a concern of the parents, the practice takes place when the child first gets home from school. Use a bridge note.

Doing a somersault across the couch when traveling from one room to another instead of walking around it.

Slamming the door or screen door when the child comes in.

Not putting school books in the back pack before going to bed.

Not emptying the dishwasher without being told.

Taking their own plates and glasses into the kitchen after they have finished eating.

Not getting dressed in the morning. This is another behavior that is practiced immediately after school or after the parent gets home. Three practices that include getting in their pajamas, waiting until the parent calls them or simulates the alarm going off, getting up, getting dressed, combing their hair, and brushing their teeth usually cure children and early adolescents of sleeping in on school mornings.

When I have informed the children who have this problem what their parents are going to have them do, I also tell them that I hope they don't get caught sleeping in anymore. About 3 out of every 10 make the mistake of not getting up on time and have to practice three times once. Only 1 out of every 10 in my clinical practice have had to practice five times. They hate it. There are too many things they want to do after school that such nonsense interferes with they say.

One mother told me that the overcorrection procedure worked so well on her 7 and 9 year old, she decided to use it on her 16 year old even though I had said there are better procedures to use with older teens. This mother got angry when she again found that her daughter had thrown clothes on the bed after trying them on instead of hanging them back on the hangers where she and her mother had placed them after ironing them. She said her daughter would try on about three outfits every morning while trying to look just right to go to school. In a hurry, she would just throw them over her head onto the bed if the outfit didn't satisfy her.

Imagine Donna's surprise when she got home from school and her mother said "follow me" and led her to the room. "Please hang up those clothes", the mother said pointing at the now somewhat wrinkled clothes laying on the bed.

"I will. I was going to do it anyway. You don't have to nag me", Donna said as she began hanging up the clothes. Mother watched

and said, "Good, that's what you should have done this morning when you took them off."

When Donna had them all hung up, her mother took them off the hangers and put them back on the bed saying, "you need practice since I've told you many times in the past to hang clothes up when you just try them on. You will practice hanging them up three times just as you watched me make your brothers put dirty clothes in the hamper three times." The mother reported that the daughter did it while grumbling, "this is stupid, stupid, stupid. You got this from that stupid Dr Marr didn't you?" Her mother also told her that the next time she didn't hang clothes up after trying them on, she would practice again. She said since then, Donna continued to say that it was stupid, but she never again left clothes laying on the bed after trying them on.

The reason why I tell parents to use other procedures with older teens is because the older they get, the more likely they are to refuse to do the practice. The parent is then left standing there insisting that the teen practice whatever and the teen saying, "Get out of my face", "No way", "I don't have to", You can't make me" or something worse. Whatever they say, we don't want to give them practice refusing to do things that the parent asks them to do. It is better to have given them positive reinforcements for the things they are doing right, such as shaping them into carrying out their responsibilities.

Although the above behavior problems are common, they cause a lot of grief for parents and children. But as the parent uses the procedures of Over-Correction, the children began to respond by remembering to pick up their clothes or put the toys away without being told. The parents began to feel calmer and the children are happier. The children are being trained to pay attention to what they are doing when the take clothes off, take their shoes off, finish riding their bicycles, etc.

CHAPTER 7

Self Control at Home and at School

The Power

Teaching children the Power has been found to be a successful method of helping them to control themselves at home and at school. This is basically a technique the child, especially one that is hyperactive, can use to quiet and calm himself in any situation. The term, "The Power", is one that the teen-agers named when they found that it gave them power over their emotions and frustrations. It is a relaxation procedure that is appropriate for the age. Usually children 6-11 can use the same procedure that is taught to the older adolescents.

In this training, the child is taught to inhale and hold his breath Then he is instructed to completely relax his face and neck when he exhales. He is encouraged to move his head a little bit when he does it. Next he takes another breath in and holds it. When he exhales, he is to relax his shoulders and arms again moving them a little. He is taught that since his arms and hands are completely relaxed, they are not to move. He then takes in a third breath and relaxes his chest, stomach, and back as he exhales. Finally he takes in the last breath and relaxes his legs and feet as he exhales.

He is cautioned to always do these parts of the body in the same order. This is done to help make the steps conditioned to his first breath. Now we must have him practice. Each afternoon or evening for the next week he is to practice twice. He is given two

points for each correct practice, one point for hurrying or being incomplete. He is told when he gets 20 points, he will be taken to an ice cream store or other place that he likes to go.

Then we must work on generalization which means we need to teach him to use it in many places including school. We want him to use his power whenever he gets excited, or frustrated, or angered. To do this we tell him that we are going to give him a 5 minute warning and then try to do something to frustrate him. When we do that, if he remembers to use his power, he gets 3 points. If he must be reminded, he only gets one. When he passes the 5 minute test two days in a row, we start giving him a 10 minute warning. "Some time in the next 10 minutes I'm going to try and frustrate you. If you remember to use your power, you get the 3 points. If I have to remind you, you only get 1 point."

When he has passed the 10 minute warning two days in a row, we give him 15 minute warnings. When he passes those tests, we began working on him to use his power in school. Some children are willing to do that on their own. But sometimes we have to tell them they will get 5 points if they come home and are able to tell us how they used their power in school.

Never force the child to do his power. If you do, they began to feel that the power is yours and not theirs. If they ever come home from school or come in from playing outside and report how they used the power in a situation, reinforce them heavily and boast about them later. That way we will get them to see that their power is rewarding as well as useful.

But we can also help them to remember use the power in school if we use the Self Instructional Training. We apply this now to encouraging the child to use his power in school.

The parent says to the child, "Pretend that the Teacher says that everybody should settle down so that you can pay attention to the lesson she is writing on the board. What should you do? You should start your power. Is that a good thing to do? Yes, because

you can better pay attention to what she is doing. Who will be happy when you do this? The Teacher is happy because you are paying attention. Your parents are happy when you pay attention in class. And most of all you will be happy because you are learning and will know what to do. Now I do the power." And the parent does the power. In fact it is a good idea if the parent uses the power at home and at work. It has been found to lower stress and blood pressure.

Notice that the parent did not ask the child to give any of the answers the first time, but instead presented a model of what the child should answer. The parent now says, "Lets do it again. Only this time you give the answers and you do the power. The Teacher says 'Alright. Everybody settle down so you can pay attention to what I am writing on the board.' What should you do?" Here the parent pauses to let the child answer. If the child doesn't answer, he is prompted and helped to get the correct response. If he must be prompted, they start over. After the child give the correct answer of saying, "I use my power.", the parent says, "Is that a good thing to do?" When the child say yes", the parent says "Why is that a good thing to do?" When the student says something to the effect of you can better pay attention to what the Teacher is writing on the board, the parent says, "Who will be happy?" And after the child says, "The Teacher, my parents, and me." Again if the child must be prompted, they start all over again, just as we described in the chapter on Self Talk. The child is also directed to use his power.

After the child gives the correct answers to all the questions, the parent says, "Very good. This time I want you to do it in a whisper, and they start over with parent prompting the child to ask the questions and give the answers. When the child can do this in a whisper, the parent says, "Now one more time only you will say it without any sound and just move your lips. And when you get to that point where you say you will be happy, give a smile

to show that you are happy as you are doing the power." The parent watches him and when the smile comes and the child does the power, the parent praises him.

I have found it helpful to tell the child that anytime he uses his power in school and then comes home and tells his parents about his use of the power, the when, where, etc, he will get 5 points and, of course, a big fuss is made over it. It doesn't take long before he is reporting regular use of the power. Points can then be thinned.

Feedback

Occasionally we find a child who learns how to use the power to quiet himself but refuses to use it at school. Sometimes that is because he enjoys the misbehavior or wants to get the attention of being a clown in school. Needless to say he is not a favorite of the teachers and he doesn't learn the material that is being taught.

Here is a solution to that problem that we have tested and found very successful. We have to tie the school behaviors more closely to after school consequences. The easiest way to do that is to send a form home daily that reports on the behaviors in school. A teacher typically has over 20 children in her room and does not have time to call every parent or write notes to every parent about the behavior of their child on a daily basis. **The School Feedback** form, shown in Table 3, was designed to make it easy for the teacher to quickly give feedback to the home and to inform the parent and the child what the feedback was.

Table 3
The School Feedback Form

Name: _____   **Date** _____

AM

Completed school work _____ + or 0.

School behavior _____ + or 0.

    Child Informed in AM _____ Teachers Initials.

PM

Completed school work _____ + or 0.

School behavior _____ + or 0.

    Child Informed in PM _____ Teachers Initials.

If the child comes home with a form that has all +'s, everybody celebrates. If the child has one 0, he loses one privilege that day. If he has two 0's he loses two privileges. If he has 3, he loses three privileges. And if he has 4 0's, he is sent to his room where he remains until bedtime. He is not allowed out even to have dinner with the family because nobody wants to eat with somebody who got 4 0's. Food is brought to the room for him to eat.

Privileges lost are such activities as TV, game playing, use of computer, going outside to play with his friends, and eating desert. Thus, if he comes home with one 0, he might then lose TV for that evening. If he has two 0's, he loses the privledge of watching TV and the privledge of playing games. And if has three 0's, he loses TV, playing games, and the privledge of going outside to play with his friends.

It is very important that the teacher know that these privileges are lost on the same day as the Feedback Form goes home. If the parent believes that the child throws the form away when there are 0's on it, the child should be informed that if he comes home

without a form, it is the same as receiving 4 0's. If the child insists that the teacher did not give him a form, then the parent must decide to call the teacher or wait until the next day and check with the teacher. If the child was telling the truth, an apology is made. If the child was not telling the truth, then he should lose the privileges on Saturday.

Typically, the use of the School Feedback Form produces a fast change in behavior at the school. Children do not like losing their fun activities at home. They began to **inhibit** inappropriate responses and try hard to get pluses. As the improvement happens, praise should increase. It also helps them to be reminded about the rules right before they get out of the car to go into the school or leave to get on the bus in the morning.

CHAPTER 8

Homework

In this chapter we will show you a major step forward in teaching ADHD children. And we do this by improving their ability and completion of their homework. Homework is a common problem of ADHD children. They forget to write down assignments, they are disorganized, they are distracted while trying to do homework, they don't want to complete the work, they are careless, and they forget to turn the work in. We have to set up a method of their doing the homework so that it is easier to monitor and easier for both child and parent.

One of the best homework programs for children who have ADHD is that called Homework Success (Power, T, Karustis, & Habboushe, 2001). It is set up to improve homework performance by improving the rates of completion of homework, the accuracy of the homework, and the efficiency of his accomplishing the assignment. The problem with that program is that it requires locating a Clinician who is qualified in the Success program knows how to lead a group of parents through the program, and it also requires a group of parents to form a team. But you don't have those and so we are going to show an alternative that is even better. It has been tested and it is successful.

In C-BAT we use similar procedures to Homework Success but we also teach the child to work in a motivated fashion. First off we must teach the child to record homework assignments so the parent knows what homework he needs to accomplish. Table 4 shows a homework assignment table that can be copied. If multiple copies

of that page are made, they can be pasted into a notebook. The parent turns to the first page and has the child copy down the date and then the names of his Subjects on the first page. He then copies down the assignments made that day in school. He then starts his homework and as he finishes each subject he crosses it out. If there was no assignment in a subject, he writes down No in that box.

For some children that instruction is all they need to start. For others we may have to use Self-Instructional Training (SIT) to get him started. SIT was illustrated in the chapter on Self-Talk. This may seem like a lot of trouble but in the long run it will save the parent time and reduce frustration.

To save you the time it takes to find it, we have repeated the instructions here. We would start out with the situation of having the child imagine that he is sitting in the classroom and the Teacher is telling everybody to copy down the homework assignment. Remember the first time we have only the parent ask and answer the questions. The parent says "What should you do? You should pull out your notebook and copy down the assignment the teacher makes. Is that a good thing to do? Yes because you will know what the assignment is when you get home. Then you can do the homework and turn it in. Who will be happy then? Your teacher, your parents and you"

Then you start over but this time your child must answer the questions. If he can't answer, you give him the answer and start all over, "Pretend that the teacher is telling everybody to copy down the homework. What should you do?" The parent pauses and waits for the child to answer. If the child doesn't say "Pull out my notebook and copy down the assignment", the parent gives him the answer and has him say it. But since you had to give him the answer, you start all over. "Pretend that the teacher says, alright everybody copy down the homework assignment. What should you do?" When he says "Pull out my notebook and copy down the assignment", the parent says "Great. Is that a good thing to do?"

and when the child says, "Yes", the parent says "Why is that a good thing to do?" and if the child doesn't answer, the parent gives him the answer and starts all over again.

When he can answer all the questions, then he must do it again, but this time he must ask and answer the questions. Thus, he must ask "What should I do?" And then answer that and ask the next question, "Is that a good thing to do?" "Yes, why is it a good thing to do?" After answering that question, we then have him do the whole thing in a whisper, and then again only moving his lips. Then finally saying it to himself. This type of exercise tells him that you will not let him escape doing the correct homework, and then turning it in. He is also learning to talk to himself.

Table 4
Homework Assignment Record

Date	Subject	Assignment

Reinforcement for Homework

Now that we have taught him to record the correct homework assignment, , we prompt the child to look at the material he has

brought home for homework and when he does, we reinforce his behavior by saying "Good" or some other term of praise. If we also give him a token, we have his attention. The token is reinforcement. He is going to be able to use his tokens to purchase activities he wants. You can use poker chips as tokens are you can make them easily out of cardboard. If you choose to make them, cut one inch by two inch coupons out of the cardboard. It is not necessary but children like them better if they are labeled as ONE on each side. You can even have the child help you make the tokens.

The list of activities that he can buy with the tokens and the cost of each in tokens is the reinforcement menu. The more attractive this menu is, the harder the child will work to get the tokens. Activities might include 30 minutes of watching TV, 30 minutes playing one of the electronic games, having Dad play catch with him, going to grandma's house, going bowling, going fishing with Dad or grandpa, having Mom play a board game with him, having a friend stay overnight, or staying at a friend's house. The more difficult it is to give him the activity or the more time it takes for the parent to give it to him, the higher the cost in tokens. It also helps if the menu is posted next to where he or she does their homework so he can see it.

He earns those tokens by doing his homework. But we are going to give him those tokens using a special procedure. We are going to reinforce him on a schedule. Schedules of reinforcement produce habits. The habit we are teaching him is to pay attention to your homework and to the work. To get the child motivated to do his homework we put him on a schedule of reinforcement. He receives a token for being on task, not for completing his work, but for <u>doing</u> the work. We have found in the Clinic that we can teach a child to work very hard on his homework if he is systematically rewarded on a schedule of reinforcement as he works. The way we do this is by starting him on a low schedule of reinforcement such as a Variable Interval of one or two minutes. These are called VI-1 or VI-2.

Sounds technical doesn't it. But we have made it easy by putting these schedules on the disks.* Simply put the first disk in the computer and start it up when the child is ready to start his homework. When he asks what the disk is for, you tell him that it is going to tell you when to reward him with a token. When he asks how, you say "Wait and see". Tell him to look at his homework again and when he does give him a token. Tell him then that he will get more tokens if he is doing the homework when the beep occurs. He will discover that when the beep occurs if he is looking at or responding to his homework, he gets one or two tokens. If he is on a VI-1 tape, he gets one token when the beep occurs and if he is on a VI-2 tape, he gets two tokens everytime the beep occurs.

Some children will want to save their tokens by banking them so that they can buy more expensive items or activities. What we do at the Clinic is give the children each a bank card. An example of a bank card is shown in Table 5.

Table 5
The Bank Card

Date	Event	Points	Balance
3-15	Homework	24	24
3-16	Homework	20	44
3-16	Spent on 30 minutes of TV	-30	14
3-17	Homework	34	48
3-17	Homework started by self	3	51
3-18	Homework	38	89
3-18	Friend Overnight	-50	39

---

* You may purchase the disks which range from VI1 to VI10 or you may make your own tapes. The times for each schedule are listed in the Appendix under **Schedules of Reinforcement.**

When the child is completed with his homework, he can count the tokens he has earned and turn them in so we can write the number of tokens he has earned, and the date they were earned on the bank card. And he can deduct tokens as he spends them. To make it easier on the parent we can even have the child keep track of the bank card and add up the points. Of course the parent will need to check and make sure the correct number of points is being added and subtracted.

The first tape used with the student is usually a **VI-1 tape** in which the beeps occur on the average of once (1) a minute. This tape delivers beeps on the average of every one minute. Sometimes it will beep after 30 seconds, after 45 seconds, after 60, after 75, after 90, etc. However, they will all occur in a random order so the child can not figure out when a beep is going to occur. But they will average out to be 1 minute apart.

When the child has reached 80% of the possible tokens on three consecutive days, she is graduated to a VI-2 tape. When she attains 80% on that tape for 3 consecutive days, she is moved to a VI-3 tape, then VI 4, VI-5, etc.

Note: When the child is on a VI-2 tape, he is to be given two tokens if he is on task when the tape beeps. Thus, if he receives two tokens after each of the 25 beeps that will occur in 50 minutes, he will have 50 tokens just as he had while on the VI-1 tape for 50 minutes. When on a VI-3 tape, he earns three tokens at each beep if on task. VI-4 beeps: four tokens; VI-5 beeps: five tokens; VI-6 beeps: six tokens, etc.

We have found that when we start a child on a VI-1 tape and move him to a higher number slowly, this produces a very steady rate of homework behavior. The children get their work done and get in the habit of turning in to the teacher the correct homework on a regular basis.

Self Talk and Self Reinforcement

It is most important that we incorporate Self Talk into our homework activities. Remember we are trying to get the children to talk to themselves about what they are doing. The more they talk to themselves the more they are using the executive function of their brains.

It is very simple to bring self talk into the homework period. All we have to do is use the beep from the VI disc to remind us. When the beep occurs, we look to see if the child is on task and if he is we give him a token. Then we say to him, "What are you doing?" If he simply says, "I'm doing my homework?", we say, "Yes but what are you doing in your homework? Are you reading, answering written questions, or are you doing addition or subtraction problems? That' what I mean when I say what are you doing? Tell me, what are you doing?"

Insist that he tell you exactly what he is doing. After you have done this a number of times he will begin to be ready to answer you by telling exactly what he is doing. That preparation to answer you, teachs him to talk to himself about his homework. "I am answering the questions about what I read." Or "I am doing my multiplication table for 7's."

We must not ask him what he is doing everytime the tape beeps but only some of the time. And not even as often as every second time. But if you ask him two or three times during every homework period, he will begin to be prepared. He is then using the executive function in his brain.

Self Esteem

Self Esteem refers to how "good" or "bad" we feel about ourselves It is our evaluation of the self. It is the ability to look at oneself and evaluate what one sees. That evaluation typically gives

rise to positive or negative feelings about the self such as pride or shame. And the positive or negative feelings are often based on how we believe others see ourselves. You can see how important this is for ADHD children. Too often they are receiving criticism from parents or teachers for their behavior.

But the other areas on which the youngsters base their evaluations are academic competence, athletic competence, social acceptance, and physical appearance. These are areas where adults can focus praise. Parents can look for things that the youngster does well in and praise him or her for these. The more that happens the more positive self worth we are creating. The more positive self worth the more we will find the child trying to receive more praise. His behavior improves.

Now consider self talk and self-esteem. We must teach him to self reinforce. We want him to be able to say to himself, "I am doing well." "Because I have been working so hard, I am almost done with my homework." To get him to say these type of things to himself we must first say them to him enough times that he begins to know what we are going to say to him. And we must prompt him to say those things. We are already occasionally asking him what he is doing while he is doing his homework. Now we must also began to say to him, "You are doing very well. Let me hear you say that. Say 'I am doing very well'" And another time "You are earning a lot of tokens. Now let me hear you say it". Push him until he begins to say positives to himself. You don't have to do this frequently but at least once every homework session. You know your child and can get him to do this. We want him to say positives to himself and often.

CHAPTER 9

Summary

We have covered a lot in this manual. We have described the characteristics of children who have ADD and ADHD. And we have described the types of treatment. Then we systematically presented the **C-BAT** to train the children to use the executive function of their brains.

The children lack self control and discipline.

The most powerful method of changing behavior is positive reinforcement.

But there is a need for discipline and a very effective type is time out.

The children need to be taught to talk to themselves.

One of the ways to help them pay attention is through over correction.

A highly successful procedure to quiet themselves is the Power.

And finally, we can teach them systematically to stay on task by using schedules of reinforcement and the token economy.

APPENDIX

Schedules of Reinforcement

For those parents who do not want to buy the tapes or discs with the schedules of reinforcement on them, we have recorded the tapes so the parents can make their own.

A sound occurs after each of the listed periods. Thus, in the Variable Interval one minute schedule, VI1 schedule, a sound would occur after 40 seconds and the next sound after one minute and 40 seconds and then after 30 seconds, etc.

The easiest way to make your own tapes is to start a tape recorder and tap a piano key or ring a bell and then start a timer. When 40 seconds have gone by, ring the bell again. Then when a minute and 40 seconds have gone by, ring the bell again, etc.

VI-1

40", 1'40", 30", 1'05", 45", 1'55", 25", 1'00", 50", 1'05", 55", 1'00", 55", 1'15", 50", 1'25", 35", 20", 1'00", 1'35", 50", 1'15", 55", 1'10", 40", 35", 1'05", 55", 30", 1'15", 35", 1'20, 50", 40", 1'45", 45", 55", 1'40", 40", 1'15", 50", 35", 1'25", 1'00", 40", 1'10", 55", 1'05", 45", 1'05", 30".

If you wish to have more times on the VI1 tape, just repeat the list above.

VI-2

1'05", 1'10", 1'15", 2'20", 1'40". 2'30", 2'00", 2'10", 1'55", 2'15", 1'45, 1'30", 1'55", 2'15", 2'10, 1'50", 2'10", 1'55", 1'55", 2'15", 1'40", 2'30".

If you wish to have more times on the VI2 tape, just repeat the list above.

VI-3

2'35", 3'15", 3'20", 3'00", 1'30", 4'15", 2'10", 4'40", 2'05", 2'50", 3'00", 2'30", 3'25", 1'35", 4,45", 2'15", 4'30, 2'50, 3'35". 3'25".

If you wish to have more times on the VI3 tape, just repeat the list above.

VI-4

30", 4'15", 3'20", 5'25", 2'10". 4'20", 3'30", 2'50", 5'15, 5'35", 2'25", 5'15", 2'10", 2'15", 3'20", 2'20", 4'55", 3'20", 2'25", 5'20", 4'30", 3'40",2'45".

V-I5

45", 3'30, 8'30", 6'00", 7'45", 3'00", 4'45", 3'15". 6'45". 5'00", 4'00", 5'30", 3'30", 4'00", 7'15", 3'05", 4'00", 3'10", 6'40", 5'05". 3'45", 7'20"

If you wish to have more times on the VI5 tape, just repeat the list above

VI-6

1'35", 4'35", 6'10", 8'40", 6'30", 9'00", 7'10", 7'00, 5'15", 4'15", 6'30", 3'10", 9'00", 4'05", 4'25", 7'15", 6'50", 5'15", 4'05", 3'15", 7'25".

VI-7

4'05", 5'50", 8'05", 9'10", 6'25", 9'05", 4'10", 10'00", 8'15", 4'20", 9'45", 5'20, 7'30".

VI-8

5'45", 11'30", 4'15", 11'05", 7'45", 12'20", 4'35", 13'30", 6'00", 5'20", 10'20, 9'15", 8'25".

VI-9

5'10", 4'30", 8'35", 14,45", 6'30", 4'50". 7'50", 15'40", 6'50", 9'00". 12'15", 5'00", 10'30".

VI-10

6'15", 11'40", 8'50", 13'15", 5'00", 14'30", 6'15", 4'15", 13'15", 7'00, 14'15", 6'05", 12'05".

REFERENCES

American Psychiatric Association. (1994). Diagnostic and statistical manual for mental disorders (4th ed.). Washington, DC: Author.

Meichenbaum, D. H.& Goodman, J. Training impulsive children to talk to themselves: a means of developing self-contol. J. Abnormal Psychology. 77, 115-126, 1971.

Power, T. J., Karustis J. L., & Habboushe, D. F. (2001). Homework Success for children with ADHD, A family-school intervention program. New York, NY. Guilford.

Made in the USA
Middletown, DE
20 October 2023

41109364R00033